I0411392

Mediterranean Diet Exposed

Foods To Burn Fat Easily Foods On The Mediterranean Diet To Drop Pounds From Day One

Kara Milanova

© 2012 by Kara Milanova

ISBN-13: 9781482608755

ISBN-10: 1482608758

First Printing, 2012

Disclaimer

This publication is intended to provide helpful and informative material. It is not intended to diagnose, treat, cure, or prevent any health problem or condition, nor is intended to replace the advice of a physician. No action should be taken solely on the contents of this book. Always consult your physician or qualified health-care professional on any matters regarding your health and before adopting any suggestions in this book or drawing inferences from it.

The author and publisher specifically disclaim all responsibility for any liability, loss or risk, personal or otherwise, which is incurred as a consequence, directly or indirectly, from the use or application of any contents of this book.

Any weight loss that may or may not occur is your responsibility and not that of the author or publisher.

Any and all product names referenced within this book are the trademarks of their respective owners. None of these owners have sponsored, authorized, endorsed, or approved this book.

Always read all information provided by the manufacturers' product labels before using their products. The author and publisher are not responsible for claims made by manufacturers.

The statements made in this book have not been evaluated by the Food and Drug Administration or any other official body.

Liability Disclaimer

By reading this book, you assume all risks associated with using the advice given below, with a full understanding that you, solely, are responsible for anything that may occur as a result of putting this information into action in any way, and regardless of your interpretation of the advice.

You further agree that our company cannot be held responsible in any way for the success or failure of your business as a result of the information presented in this book. It is your responsibility to conduct your own due diligence regarding the safe and successful operation of your business if you intend to apply any of our information in any way to your business operations.

Terms of Use

You are given a non-transferable, "personal use" license to this book. You cannot distribute it or share it with other individuals.

Also, there are no resale rights or private label rights granted when purchasing this book. In other words, it's for your own personal use only.

Mediterranean Diet Exposed

Foods To Burn Fat Easily Foods On The Mediterranean Diet To Drop Pounds From Day One

Table of Contents

1 - The Benefits of Eating Mediterranean

Everyone wants a life that if free of any suffering and disease. With all the challenges that we face with modern living like processed foods and stress it is a bit hard to achieve. Despite all this people that live in the **Mediterranean** have benefited from greater overall health and higher life expectancy.

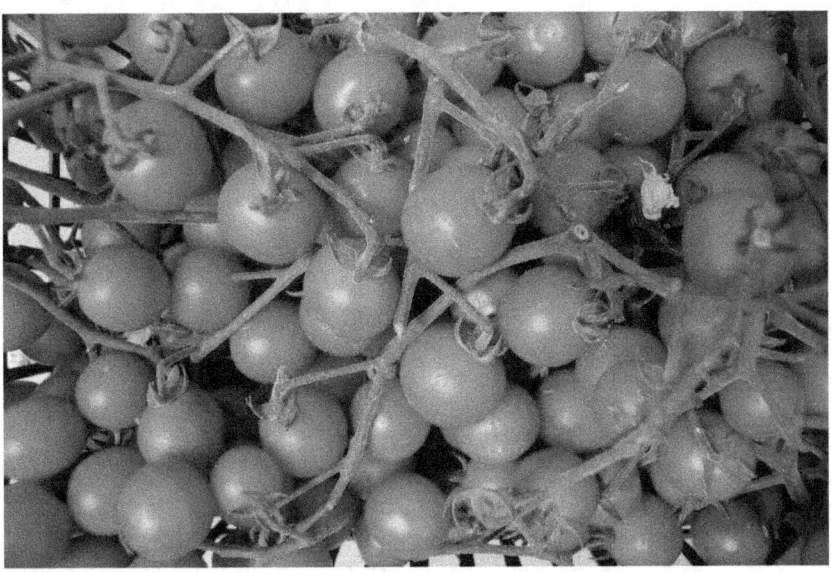

This is basically due to the foods that they consume. They eat lots of plant based foods like vegetables, fruits, legumes, nuts and whole grains. Instead of red meat they eat a lot of fish and indulge in a little red wine with most meals. The food does have a high fat content but it is monounsaturated fatty acid (olive oil) that is beneficial for heart health. The peoples of the Mediterranean who eat a traditional diet tend to live longer and have fewer health problems.

One of the major benefits of the Mediterranean diet is that it is great for cardiac health. Studies that have been conducted on people living in the Mediterranean have shown that they have lower levels of heart disease than the rest of the world. In fact a study conducted all the way back in nineteen ninety five had shown that people with cardiac problems that were placed in the Mediterranean diet had fewer incidences of heart attacks (*approximately seventy percent*). It was also noted that their LDL cholesterol levels, triglyceride and blood pressure had stabilized significantly. This does not come as a surprise as the diet has a lot of monounsaturated fatty acids that are great for heart health. The next benefit is that it also helps stave off type II diabetes by helping to keep the hypo glycemic levels low.

Yet another benefit of being on this diet is the prevention of cancer. In Greece and other countries cancer is not as prevalent as it is in say the United States. This is a result of the high levels of vegetables and fruits that are consumed on a regular basis. It is well known that these food items are full of antioxidants which help to fight off free radicals that can cause mutations in the cells leading to cancer. The high fiber content helps to protect the bowel. Eating tomatoes, especially if they are cooked is thought to be particularly good for men as it offers some protection from testicular cancer. Superb tomatoes are grown in the Mediterranean region and used frequently in cooked dishes and in salads.

Last but not least the diet has many more benefits than the physical. In a study it revealed that the high consumption of legumes, nuts and fruits are essential in cutting down the risk of depression. Being on this diet may also help reduce the incidences of Parkinson's and Alzheimer's. Even the slightest modifications like a switch to using olive oil instead of the other types of fats will be beneficial.

2 - Olive Oil and Other Fats: What You Need to Know

Olives are the source of olive oil and are a traditional crop in the Mediterranean. A lot of producers that make olive oil are found in North Africa, Southern Europe and the Near East. In Europe the major producers are Greece, Portugal and Spain. The source of the oil is dependent on the type of crop and the source of the seed.

Fat Consumption and Calories

Considered one of the healthiest oils to use for cooking this oil is made up of approximately seventy three percent monounsaturated fat and fourteen percent saturated fat. A table spoon of olive oil contains approximately one hundred and twenty calories.

Other vegetable oils have varying percentages of polyunsaturated, monounsaturated and saturated fats. Coconut oil contains approximately ninety two percent saturated fats, and is typically used as shortening and in desserts. Other oils like sunflower and canola oil contain higher levels of monounsaturated fat (eighty two and sixty two percent) and is a better choice for use second to olive oil. Of course depending on the source of the data the figures will vary.

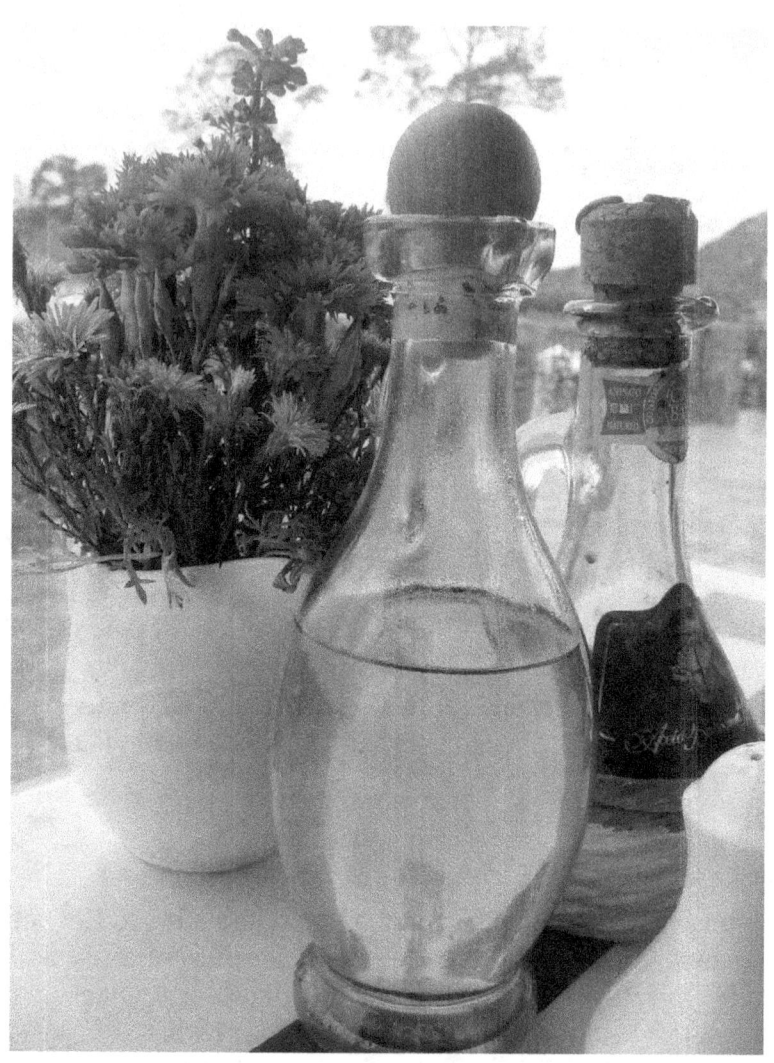

Uses

Olive oil is great for the skin, can be used for cooking and has some medicinal properties as well. It can be used as a laxative and is also used to prepare various medications. In a number of religions like Judaism and Christianity olive oil symbolizes healing.

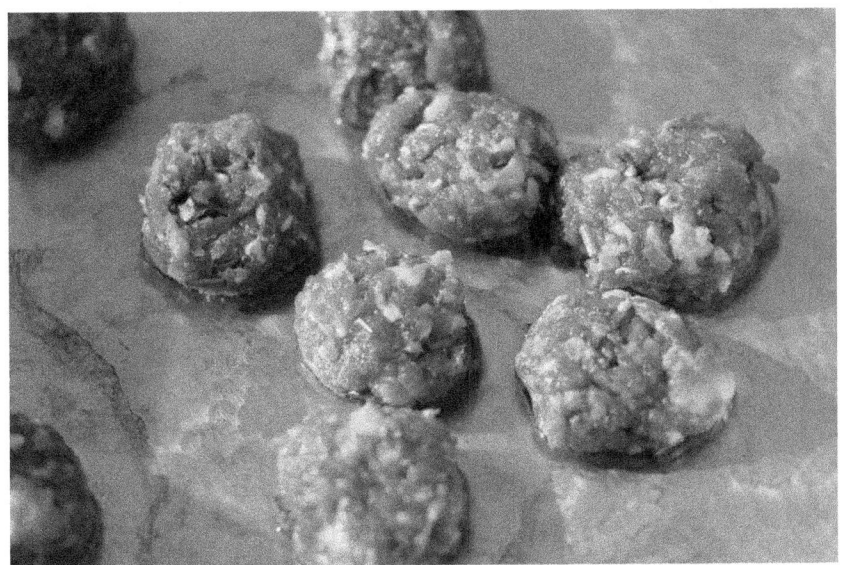

Even though vegetable oils are mostly used for cooking, they can also be used to make cosmetics, fuel, medicine and also serve other purposes.

Types

There are three kinds of olive oil pure, virgin and extra virgin. The most expensive option is the extra virgin. This is made from the first cold press and has the lowest level of free fatty acids of the three types (less than one percent). As it has the best color and aroma it is served with bread and used in dressings. For most of us it is difficult to detect the subtle differences in the oil caused by the weather, soil and aspect of the olive grove but experts can tell the region of origin and the year of pressing. Extra virgin oil is as distinctive as wine.

The second type of oil, virgin, is made by pressing the olives a second time but has a higher level of free fatty acids (around 2%). The last type is a blend of refined olive oil and virgin oil usually labeled "Pure Olive Oil" or just "Olive Oil". It is not as expensive and is typically used for high temperature cooking. Light and refined olive oil goes through chemical processing to get rid of strong tastes and produce a more standardized product. The health benefits are not affected by the chemical processing although it may have a slightly higher free fatty acid level.

The grading system used in the USA is very similar to that used by Mediterranean producers.

US Extra Virgin Olive Oil has a free fatty acid content of no more than 0.8%

US Virgin Olive Oil has a free fatty acid content of no more than 2%

US Olive oil is a mixture of virgin and refined oils.

The grades are voluntary.

Arizona, California and Texas have all started to produce olive oil and the oil is now beginning to be stocked in supermarkets.

Other types of vegetables oils include rice bran oil, sesame oil, grape seed oil, peanut oil, safflower oil, sunflower oil, corn oil, pumpkin seed oil, canola oil, soya bean oil and palm oil. Sunflower oil is used quite widely in the Mediterranean region as it is cheaper than olive oil and it is healthier than animal fats.

Properties

The temperature at which the oil starts to burn is known as the smoke point. Light oils are best for high temperature cooking. Olive oil has a lower smoke point than other types of vegetable oil and varies from two hundred and fifteen degrees and two hundred and forty two degrees. The lighter version of olive oil has a higher smoke point than extra virgin olive oil.

Benefits for Health

Olive oil is a rich source of minerals and vitamins based on how it was processed. It is thought to help reduce the instances of heart disease as a result of the high level of monounsaturated fatty acids like oleic acids. This helps to increase the levels of HDL and decrease the levels of LDL and makes the arterial walls more elastic. It has antioxidant properties that help to cut down on the amount of cholesterol in the blood.

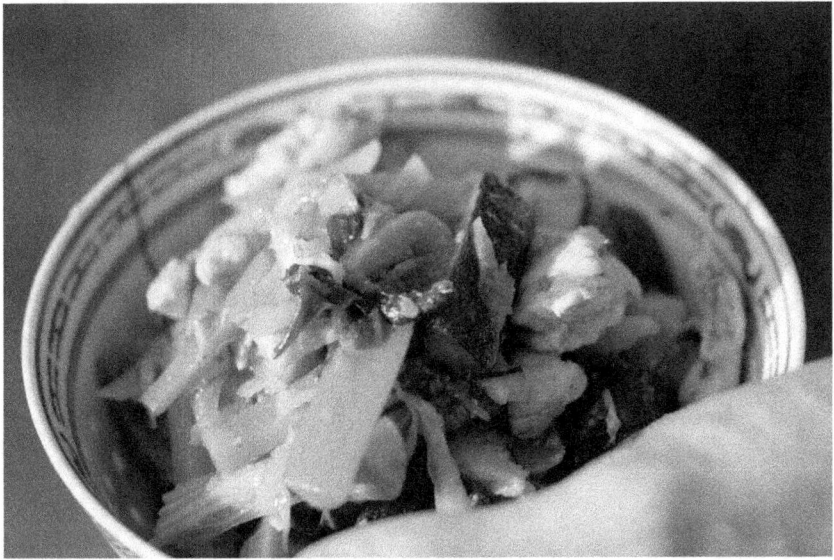

Some vegetable oils help to lower the amount of saturated fat and are not as expensive as olive oil but there is a certain amount of evidence that canola oil has some negative health properties and probably should be avoided. Other types of oils like coconut oil and sesame oil are used in small quantities to flavor dishes.

Garlic

Garlic is used widely throughout Mediterranean countries to give depth and flavor to the food. If you really hate garlic then just leave it out of recipes. If you are willing to give it a go then start by adding just a single clove – that is one segment of the garlic bulb. When your palate is accustomed to this you can try adding a little more.

Garlic is thought to lower blood pressure, lower cholesterol levels, protect against strokes and to fight infections. Studies suggest that this might well be the case. Records for the medicinal use of garlic go back 5000 years to India.

People today take garlic to prevent colds and many say that it works well for them. If you include it in your cooking you could be reaping extra benefit from your Mediterranean life style.

3 - Vegetables: The Heart and Soul of the Traditional Mediterranean Diet

One of the best things about this type of diet is that the foods can be found quite easily. The bulk of the diet consists of seeds, rice, pasta, nuts, beans, whole grains, vegetables and fruits. Unlimited amounts of vegetables can be eaten and no vegetable is taboo. To add some flavor to the vegetables they can be lightly sautéed with some olive oil. With all the choices there are you will never be bored with your food.

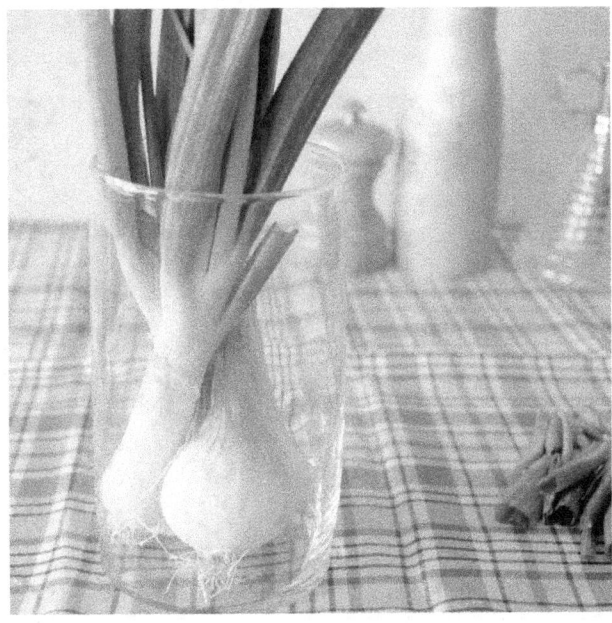

Focus on High Fiber

Selecting vegetables with high fiber content will improve the health of the digestive system and the heart. The vegetable with the highest level of fiber are peas and beans which can be sautéed with some fresh tomatoes and scallions in some olive oil to make a perfect Mediterranean diet recipe. Spinach which is also high in fiber can be eaten raw as part of a salad, added to pasta sauces or cooked on its own. Squash or zucchini make great choices as well.

Vegetables with Antioxidants

When you opt to go on the Mediterranean diet, select vegetables that help stave off diseases like heart disease and cancer. A lot of vegetables are filled with antioxidants that help to combat the effects of free radicals on the cells in the body. Orange, dark green, red and other brightly colored vegetables are full of antioxidants. Tomatoes, dark green leafy vegetables and orange and red bell peppers are just a few of these power packed vegetables. As the dishes frequently use olive oil in preparation the level of antioxidants that the body gets is increased.

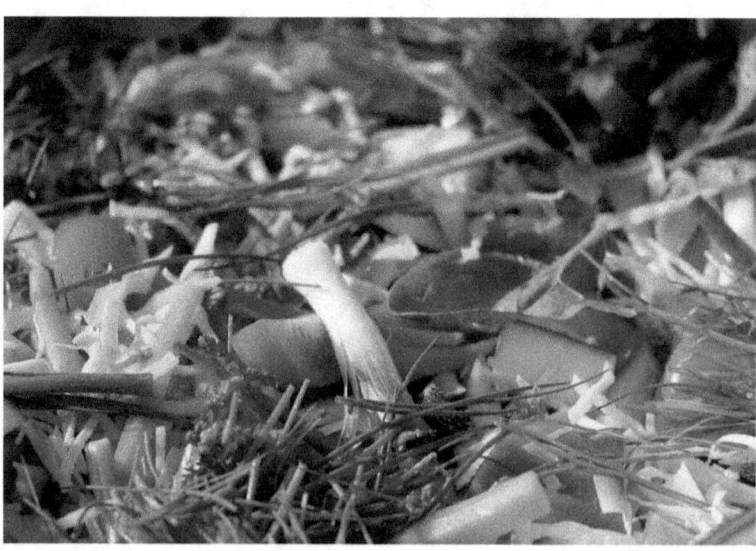

Try New Things

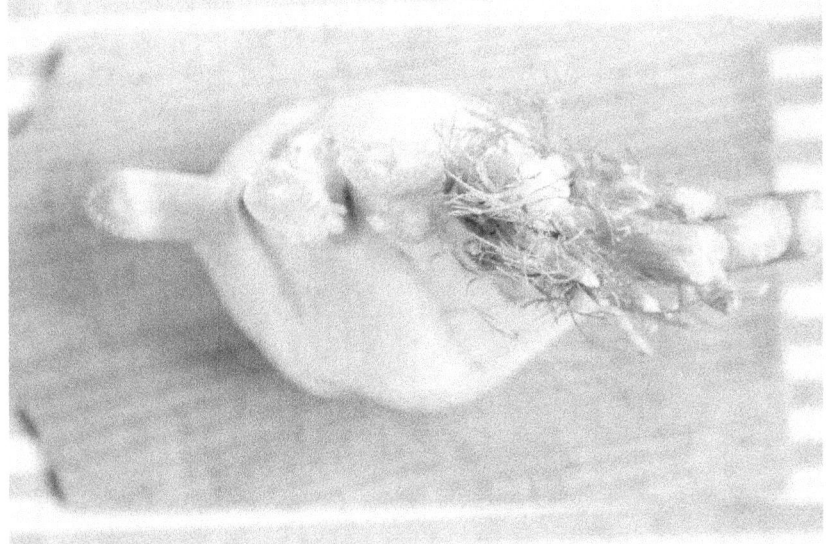

The vegetables from the Mediterranean may seem a bit strange to you but they come packed with loads of fiber and nutrients and taste delicious. They will help you to lose weight as you set out on the path to a healthier lifestyle.

A vegetable that is commonly used is eggplant (aubergine). It can simply be sliced up, seasoned and sautéed in some olive oil. You can leave the skin on if you want-nothing is simpler. A typical dish is to sauté the eggplant with a little garlic and serve it over some pasta. Many people love it for the distinctive yet not overwhelming flavor.

4 - The Fruits of Good Health

Some may wonder what all the hype is about when it comes to eating all this fruit. It is not only healthier but can help with weight loss, and the cleansing of the body. It can also help in maintaining weight at healthy levels. Fruit gives the benefits of high fiber content along with vitamins and minerals. Oranges ,for instance, have a high level of vitamin C which is essential for health and cannot be stored in the body. You should remember that fruits and some vegetables do contain natural sugars which are as fattening as any other sugar. If your aim is weight loss you might need to strike a balance here. Fruit is much better for you than very sugary or fatty foods and obviously less fattening but maybe you would not want to eat unlimited quantities.

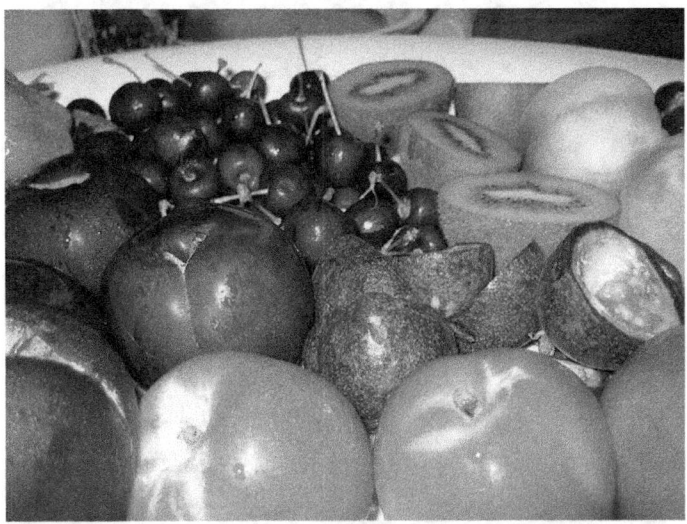

<u>Fruity Facts!</u>

Cholesterol free

High percentage of water, just like the human body

May improve memory

Improves the way one feels

Full of great healing properties, vitamins and essential minerals

Full of fiber

Very tasty

As stated before, the majority of fruit is made up of water. If you think about it the theory does seem sound to have foods that contain a lot of water like the body.

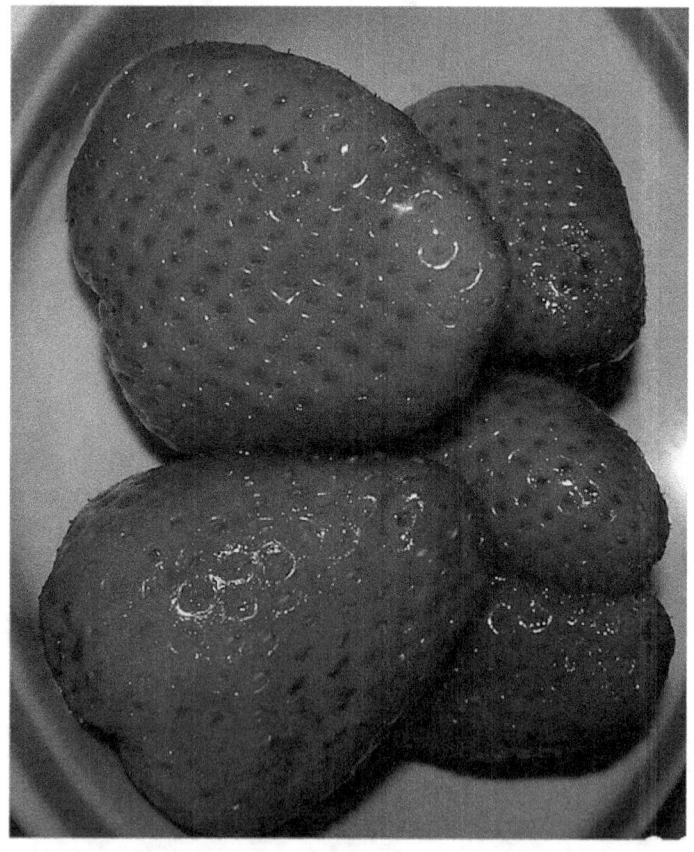

Fruit and vegetables are so good for you that they form the

major part of the diet for vegetarians and especially vegans.

There can be no disputing the fact that fruit contains no cholesterol at all. It is well known that cholesterol is not good for us. Things we consume daily like dairy and meat contain a lot of bad cholesterol.

Fruits have also been suggested as good fuel for the brain as they work well to stimulate the memory. Research continues to find out just how it all works. It is thought that people who consume a lot of fruit tend to have better memory recall.

The healing effects that fruits have are also being noticed. For example seamen on long voyages in sailing ships used to suffer and die from a disease called scurvy. The English Captain Cook insisted that his sailors had half a lime every day and not one of his men fell ill from scurvy. It was discovered that the vitamin C in the limes prevented the disease. This is where the name some Americans use for English people, "limey", comes from. Not all the health benefits of fruit eating can be illustrated so dramatically!

Now lets us look at the fiber content. It is well known that a diet filled with fiber helps with hypertension, obesity speeds digestive transit. The level of fiber that is consumed is very useful in helping to ensure a healthy digestive system.

It cannot be disputed that fruit is a natural food. One can easily pick a fruit from a tree eat it and dispose of the seed. This keeps the cycle of life going for the particular fruit and keeps the body healthy.

The healthiest diet is made up of vegetables, raw fruits and freshly squeezed fruit juices, along with some protein and carbohydrate. A few tips are outlined below.

It works in your favor to start drinking fresh fruit juices (and water) and eating raw fruits.

Fruits work best if consumed on an empty stomach and not after a meal is consumed.

One will feel better after staring to eat fruits regularly. Aim for at least five portions of fruit or vegetables every day as a minimum amount.

5 - The Grains, Legumes, Nuts, and Seeds of the Mediterranean

Seeds, nuts, legumes and grains can be considered the body of Mediterranean cuisine. This makes up the bulk of the traditional diet and the many types of seeds, nuts, legumes and grains help to make filling, fragrant and wonderfully satisfying food.

The smell of freshly baked bread is a distinguishing factor in a Mediterranean kitchen. It could be a Moroccan flatbread or country bread or round bread from France, the fact is that whole grain bread is served with most Mediterranean meals in some form. Pannini and bruschetta are popular forms of Italian bread that have become fashionable in recent years.

Can you just see all types of pasta from tagliatelle to orecchiette (little ears) and rice shaped orzo, giant shells or even lasagna steaming in pots? This is the sort of thing that can be found on the tables of Italy. Couscous, a semolina made from duram wheat, is more popular in countries on the Southern shores of the Mediterranean, like Morocco. All the Mediterranean countries have their favorite forms of carbohydrate that give people stamina for their working day. The traditional diet was evolved by people who did a heavy days work in the fields without the help of modern machinery so most people do not need the big helpings of carbohydrates . Enjoy the pasta or the bread but watch the portion size. Be adventurous and enjoy the different shapes of pasta and different sauces to go with them, Pasta shapes like bows or

31

shells hold the sauce better than the long thin shapes like sphaggetti.

A great variety of vegetables can be used in a popular Italian recipe known as creamy risotto. Other rice dishes are popular as well like Greek rice pilaf or saffron colored Spanish rice used for Spanish paella and a whole host of other combinations of rice with seafood or vegetables can be found in recipe books.

Another great Italian specialty is cornmeal based polenta; it is porridge like when it is fresh and can be sliced and grilled when chilled. Another specialty are the Italian dumplings known as gnocchi made from flour. If we journey to the Middle Eastern shores we will find bulgur wheat which is used in tabouli salad and pilafs. Of course the moussaka, meat and vegetable pies, calzone and pizza cannot be left out.

Grains are found at the base of the pyramid in the Mediterranean diet. This means that there are two or three servings of polenta, couscous, bulgur, rice, cereal, pasta, whole grain breads and other things each day. So, one of the best ways to adopt the Mediterranean style of eating is to incorporate more whole grains in your diet.

The grains can have interesting and tasty additions like seeds, nuts and protein rich legumes. Spaghetti with walnut sauce, chickpeas with bulgur wheat, rice with peas, and penne with white beans are examples. Legumes are grown in every country in the Mediterranean and often replace meat in the main course or help to stretch meals with meat so that a little goes a long way.

Legumes are rich in fiber and protein, minerals (like selenium) and vitamins (like folacin). They come in a variety of colors, sizes and types and some of the common ones are Egyptian full beans, lima beans, red kidney beans, tiny white haricot beans, red and green lentils, black beans, broad beans, garbanzo beans and white cannelloni beans. They can be eaten with a a splash of lemon juice and a little olive oil.

A lot of cultures have used legumes for centuries as a major source of protein and in the Mediterranean this is no exception.

Seeds and nuts are used to add crunch and flavor to cooked and raw foods. They could be an appetizer (hummus with almond paste mixed with chickpeas, main course (a pasta and pesto containing loads of pine nuts) or dessert (nuts sprinkled over stewed fruit).

Seeds and nuts contain significant nutrients, monounsaturated fats, protein and phytochemicals typical to the Mediterranean diet. Though a lot of the seeds and nuts have a high fat content, only approximately ten percent of the fat is saturated fat.

Consuming seeds and nuts on a regular basis has been linked to low incidences of a number of chronic illnesses like some heart diseases and cancers. Although these foods have health benefits they should be eaten in moderation. Fats still have a high calorific value even if they are unsaturated. If you are interested in weight loss use nuts as a substitute for other high calorie foods rather than have them as extra snacks. Some roasted nuts are very high in fat. Just notice how greasy you hands are after handling them.

Nuts, peanuts, pistachios, pine nuts, hazelnuts, almonds and walnuts are typically found in this part of the world. Other kinds of seeds and nuts that you might want to experiment with include sunflower seeds, sesame seeds, pumpkin seeds, pecans, cashews and chestnuts.

The main thing to bear in mind is that all seeds and nuts with the exception of coconut can be incorporated into the Mediterranean diet. One would just have to ensure that these seeds and nuts are not packaged with hydrogenated oils or trans-fatty acids.

Seeds and nuts whether roasted or plain and without added salt and oils are a great snack food. Dried fruits like blueberries, dried cherries, dates, currants, raisins and so on are also great nutritious snacks between meals.

6 - Meat, Poultry, Fish, Dairy, and Egg Consumption the Mediterranean Way

In this particular diet plan meat is not consumed on a daily basis. Meat is typically had three to four times per week.

Red Meat- in the typical Mediterranean diet red meat is rarely eaten. It is consumed on special occasions and no more than a few times per month. Red meat refers to lamb a traditional Easter dish and ground beef cooked in Moussaka and other dishes.

Poultry and Eggs- poultry is a popular meat in the diet with chicken being the most common. Quail and duck are also consumed. Eggs are not eaten on a daily basis but can be used for breakfast.

As has been stated before throughout this book, this diet is great for heart health. Recent studies have revealed that a Mediterranean diet that includes a lot of omega 3 rich, oily fish helps lower the risk of diabetes, metabolic syndrome, stroke and heart disease. Consuming more fish (like salmon and sardines) can help longevity.

Metabolic syndrome, a condition that is on the rise in certain countries occurs when as individual has a combination of the symptoms below:

Good cholesterol HDL that is lower than 50 in women and 40 in men

Fasting blood sugar that is more than one hundred mg per dL

Triglyceride count higher that one hundred and fifty per dL

Blood pressure that is more than 130/85

A waist measurement that is greater than 40 inches for men and 35 inches for women.

Research and Omega 3 Fish Oil

After going through the results of in excess of fifty scientific studies, researchers in Italy and Greece have come to the conclusion that a diet rich in fish improves the ratio of good cholesterol (HDL) to bad cholesterol (**LDL**), lowers triglycerides, blood sugar and blood pressure. The results of the study were published by the American College of Cardiology.

Oily fish is anecdotally linked to improved memory and to joint mobility.

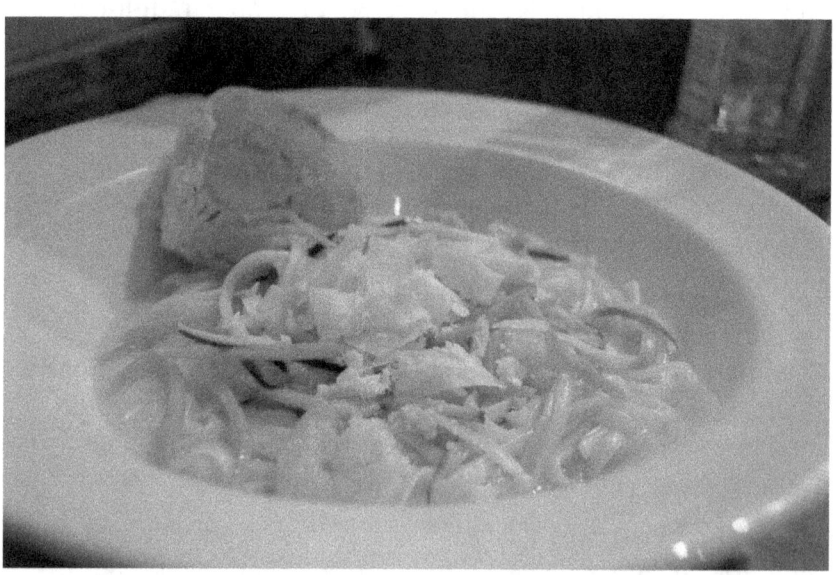

A great Mediterranean diet will have daily servings of low fat dairy products, whole grain cereals, fruits, vegetables and also include weekly portions of seeds, nuts, beans poultry and fish.

It also incorporates the use of monounsaturated olive oil along with moderate consumption of wine that is had with meals. The consumption of red meat and processed foods are restricted. This is because, historically, the peasants could not afford much meat and could only eat what they reared themselves. Consequently they did not eat beef as cattle take up a lot of space and need a lot of fodder, Most people had space for a few chickens and maybe a goat. Traditionally people ate food they grew themselves so very little was processed in the modern sense.

Fish with high levels of omega 3 fatty acids like trout, herring, sardines and salmon are great for lessening the possibility of having metabolic syndrome. It is great for the cardiovascular system. It is also essential for early childhood brain development including infancy and foetal stages. It can help stave off some eye problems. In adults it is thought that it might also help with Alzheimer's disease, depression and arthritis.

Most dietary guides recommend that a portion of oily fish be consumed at least two or more times during the week. This can be difficult especially if you live some way from the sea as really fresh fish is hard to get. Although the omega 3 will survive freezing and canning the fish is not quite as tasty as it would be were it freshly caught. It is well worth making the effort to include oily fish in your diet and if you buy from a reputable source you do not have to worry about toxicity as this is only an issue in a few parts of the world where seas are heavily polluted by industrial waste. If you are worried about fish toxicity it likely that having fish rich in omegas 3 two or three times per week is much more beneficial than any side effect. To keep the risk of toxicity down avoid eating fish like tilefish, king mackerel, shark and swordfish.

Types

Dairy products are used in this diet in moderation as in most hot countries. Yogurt, cheese and milk can be consumed on their own or as part of other dishes. In a few cultures on the

Mediterranean coast milk from buffalo, sheep and goats are used instead of cow's milk. The mozzarella cheese traditionally used on pizza in Italy is made from buffalo milk. Parmesan cheese is used sprinkled on many dishes. Although it has a high fat content it is very strong and used very sparingly. It is best to have low fat dairy products whenever possible even though some full fat products can be enjoyed in moderation.

People in this region tend to eat less dairy than people in North America. Olive oil and nuts which are plant based lipids are the major source of dietary fat. People on this type of diet can consume one serving of dairy per day while others can have milk products on a weekly basis. Eggs are not eaten often either and should not be eaten more than four times per week.

Fallacies

Mediterranean foods with an American flair have more dairy than the traditional diet. An American pizza, for example, has lots of cheese when compared to the classic Italian pizzas which may have very little or no cheese at all. Olive oil is used instead of butter and full fat dairy is rarely consumed.

Advantages

When consumed in moderation milk products have nutritional benefits. These products have naturally occurring calcium, dietary protein and some have micronutrients like vitamin D. in addition to that, products like yogurt and buttermilk (cultured dairy products) contain probiotics which are also known as friendly bacteria. Full fat dairy products work better for people that are underweight as it provides a mega source of dietary calories. Young children need calcium for the development of strong bones and teeth and should be given dairy products in sensible amounts for their size and age.

Disadvantages

Health benefits can be linked to the limited use of dairy products. Milk products tend to be rich in saturated fat and can increase the risk of cardiovascular problems by combating bad cholesterol and triglyceride levels. It is recommended that no more than two servings of milk based products should be consumed per day. Use half fat milk or skimmed milk which has only a trace of fat as alternatives. If you have heart disease it is helpful to follow the traditional Mediterranean diet.

7 - Embracing the Mediterranean Lifestyle

What is it that makes the Mediterranean lifestyle and diet so great?

Why do people in this region live happier and longer lives?

There are a number of reasons for that but the one outlined below are the most important:

Fresh food on a daily basis

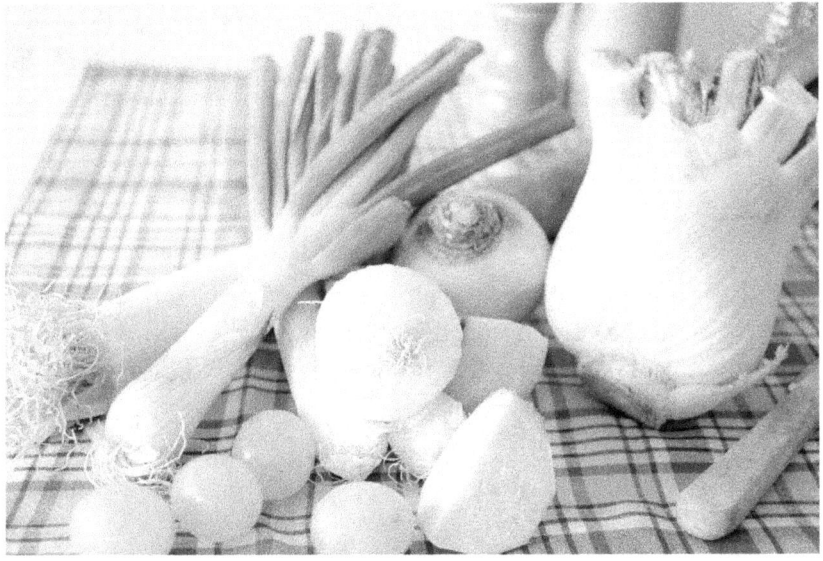

Most towns, and even villages, have markets which provide fresh olive oil, seeds, nuts, pulses, meat, fish, salads, vegetables and fruit. People go to the market and interact. Food is very important to these people and they are very passionate about it. It is more than just getting fuel for the body. They go through the market tasting, smelling and touching the food before they make a purchase. They want the best items to make their meals. The market acts as a commercial and social center of the Mediterranean life.

Family Values

This is something that is fading fast in some societies. People in this region have a deep value for the family and everything it entails. The family does everything together and can often be seen working together. A typical French family can be seen having a picnic at a table filled with crusty bread, charcuterie, fresh salads and of course wine. The Italian family will be dining together having grilled fish and meat, foccacia bread, salads and pasta.

Slow Down – Get Out of the Fast Lane for A Minute

Take a look at this culture and learn from it. They take time to relax and really enjoy what life has to offer. Spend an afternoon eating a fresh salsa verde with grilled swordfish steak and sipping a chilled Rosé or have a pizza made in a wood burning oven. The secret is to slow down and savor it all. Take some time to just indulge. It will work wonders for the stress you build up rushing about all day.

That is basically it- get in the slow lane once in a while. Take a trip to the market to get your fresh produce and just take some time to relax with the family- it does not get any better than that.

8 - Losing Weight and Living Well on the Mediterranean Diet

The Mediterranean diet is pretty easy to follow as the selection of foods is full of flavorful fats, beans, seeds, nuts, vegetables, fruits, cereals and whole breads and a lot of other foods that stave off hunger. The most beneficial aspect of this diet is the fact that it is rather effective at triggering weight loss especially in the abdominal area.

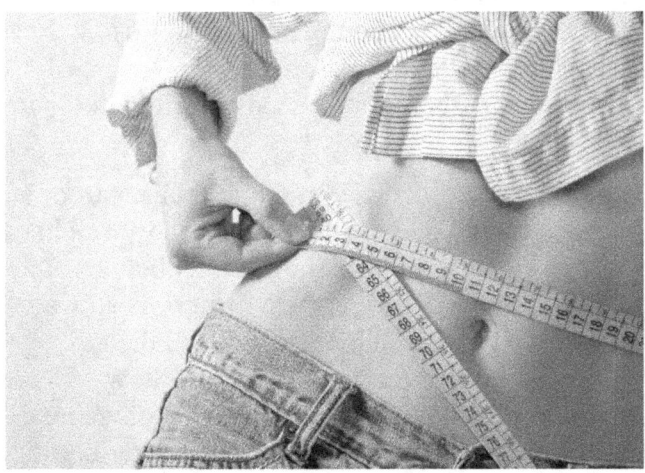

When you are overweight it can really make a difference in how healthy you are. Having too much fat in the abdominal area can cause crowding of the internal organs and this sets off a chain reaction of negative things that impact health. It can range from an increase in bad cholesterol (LDL) to heart disease, diabetes and high blood pressure.

If you get a tape measure and get the measurement by placing it just above the hip bones you will know where you stand. It if is more than thirty five inches if you are female and more than forty inches if you are male you need to make some changes to your diet quickly. The answer lies in the Mediterranean diet.

The Mediterranean way of eating will only work as a weight loss diet if you eat in moderation. Whatever diet you choose you will only loose weight by eating less. There is no magic fix. The foods in the Mediterranean way of eating have benefits whatever your size or shape and with an immense variety to choose from you need not find it boring or feel deprived. Whole grains are more filling than refined flours so you will not want to eat so much. You can fill up on fruit and vegetables which are better for you than sugar and fat laden deserts. Use a simple recipe book (and don't forget the recipes in the next chapter of this book) and try to cook most things from basic ingredients. Store bought pizzas, for example, have a high fat content. The more you cook the easier and quicker it becomes. It is satisfying to cook your own food and once you are in the habit it helps you to slow down and relax. You are less likely to gobble your meal down quickly so you are more aware of the messages of fullness that your body sends and less likely to overeat.

You will not loose weight rapidly as you might at the start of a fad diet, but the changes you make will lead to steady weight loss. As this new way of eating will make you feel better you will find it easier to continue eating in the Mediterranean way and carry on loosing weight over a long period and then to sustain your preferred weight over the long term. Allow yourself an occasional treat, just do not make every day a treat day! It is really just dietary common sense and moderation. If you overeat one day it is not disaster as long as you go back to more moderate eating the day after.

As in all weight loss regimes you do need to exercise a little to use some of the calories you eat and to speed up metabolism. Exercise also suppresses appetite so it is an all win scenario. Choose a form of exercise that suits you and your lifestyle and have several sessions each week. Walking is often the easiest way to exercise within the framework of your normal life.

9 - Recipes for Enjoying the Mediterranean Diet

Rich in culture and food history, the nations on the shores of the brilliant azure Mediterranean Sea—Italy, Spain, France, Morocco, Greece, Lebanon, Syria, Turkey and Israel—have all contributed something special to the colorful, vibrant tapestry that is Mediterranean cuisine.

Key components of Mediterranean cuisine include heart-healthy olive oil, protein-rich legumes, fish and whole grains with moderate amounts of wine and red meat. The flavors are rich, and the health benefits for people choosing a Mediterranean diet are hard to ignore—they are less likely to develop high blood pressure, high cholesterol or become obese.

This collection features delicious and nourishing recipes that evoke the essence of the Mediterranean region while helping you work your way toward optimal health.

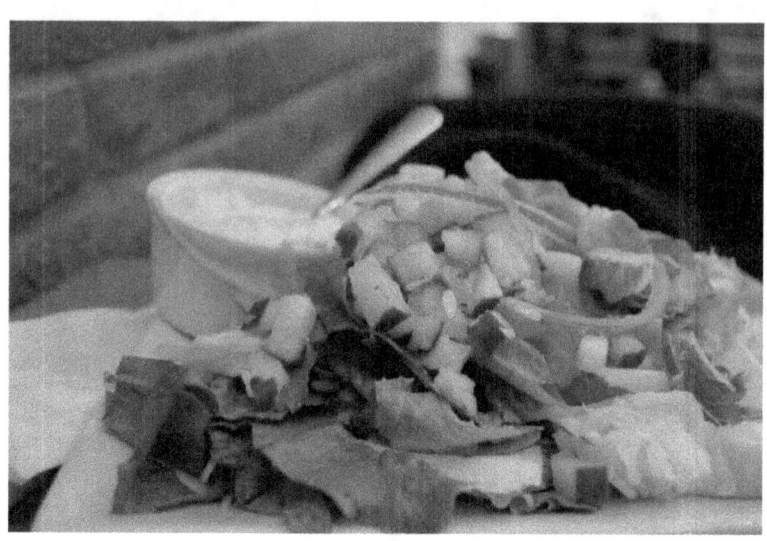

<u>Basic Tomato Sauce for Use in Pasta or Rice Dishes</u>

This sauce is a great standby for a quick and simple meal and it can be frozen in portions for use when you are short of time or too tired to bother much.

Makes 21/4 pints or 5 cups

Ingredients

4 tablespoons olive oil

1 large onion , chopped

4 cloves of garlic, crushed (that is 4 of the little segments of a garlic bulb not 4 whole bulbs)

13 oz can chopped tomatoes

1lb ripe fresh tomatoes peeled

(An easy way to peel tomatoes --- prick them all over with the tip of a pointed knife, put in a bowl and cover in boiling water, stand for 10 minutes, place in cold water then the skins should come off easily)

4 tablespoons chopped parsley

1 pint / 2 1/2 cups hot vegetable stock

1 tablespoon of sugar

2 tablespoons of lemon juice

¼ pint of dry white wine (optional) or extra stock

salt and pepper

Method

Heat the oil in a large saucepan and add the onion and garlic. Fry for about 3 minutes until they start to soften.

Add canned and fresh tomatoes, parsley stock and lemon juice. Bring to the boil and stir well. Cover the pan and simmer for 15 minutes,

Stir in the wine and seasoning then taste and just the seasoning if necessary. If it is too acidic add a little more sugar.

At this point set aside any sauce that you intend to freeze or to store in your refrigerator (will keep for 5 days)

Now add any pieces of cooked meat , fish or raw, sliced mushroom to the remaining sauce, bring it back to the simmer and cook for a few minutes longer.

Pour over pasta or rice and serve with a sprinkle of Parmesan cheese.

This sauce can be served plain, without any additions, for a very simple meal. You might like a little more Parmesan in this case.

Butternut Squash Pilaf

Butternut squash that is grated adds nutrients and color to rice pilaf. The Greeks like to use pumpkin and other winter squash to make sweet and savory pies, croquettes and fritters and many other dishes.

Ingredients

3 tablespoons extra virgin olive oil

2 pounds (peeled, halved and seeded) butternut squash

1 large finely chopped red onion

2 tablespoons water

1 clove garlic, minced

1 cup parboiled or instant brown rice

1 tablespoon tomato paste

½ cup white wine

1 ¾ cups water or one fourteen ounce can of vegetable broth

½ cup fennel fronds (chopped)

1 teaspoon salt

2 tablespoons fresh oregano (chopped)

Freshly ground pepper (to taste)

Pinch of cinnamon

Method

Using the large side of the grater, grate the squash.

Heat oil in a nonstick or cast iron skillet using medium heat then add garlic and onions and allow to cook until they are lightly colored and soft. This should take ten to twelve minutes. Mix tomato paste with two tablespoons water and then add to the pan. Add the squash and stir until the pan can be covered.

Turn the heat up to medium high and add one and three quarter cups wine and broth then cover and allow to come to a broil. Turn the heat down and stir occasionally until the rice has soaked up most of the liquid and the squash is tender (twenty five to thirty minutes).

Add the pepper, cinnamon, salt, and oregano and fennel fronds and stir to mix. Take off the stove and allow to stand for five minutes. Serve at room temperature or hot.

Warm Arugula Bread Salad

This panzanella is best when made with arugula that is mature but baby arugula can be used as well. It can be served with turkey sausage or cold roast chicken.

Arugula has many names but is one of the rocket family and any type of rocket may be used

Ingredients

2 slices crusty whole-wheat bread (cut into one inch cubes)

3 tablespoons divided extra-virgin olive oil

7 ounces arugula

1 cup halved cherry tomatoes

1/8 teaspoon salt

1 tablespoon garlic (minced)

2 tablespoons vinegar (balsamic)

¾ ounce shaved or grated Parmesan cheese

Method

In a large skillet, heat two tablespoons of oil. Add bread and stir until it starts to brown and is crisp. Add arugula and tomatoes and continue to stir occasionally until arugula wilts. Push ingredients to one side and add remaining oil to the empty side of the pan and cook the garlic until it is sizzling and fragrant. Mix all ingredients in pan then remove it from the heat and season with pepper and salt, add some vinegar and toss to mix. Serve warm with some Parmesan on top.

Chicken & Farfalle with Creamy Walnut Sauce

Ingredients

1 small peeled clove garlic

Salt (¼ teaspoon)

1/3 cup walnuts

Cayenne pepper (pinch)

¼ teaspoon pepper (freshly ground)

2 tablespoons fresh parsley (finely chopped)

¼ cup chicken broth (reduced sodium)

Lemon juice (½ teaspoon)

8 ounces fat free chicken breast (boneless & skinless), cut into ½ inch portions

½ red bell pepper (cut into thin strips and seeded)

1 teaspoon extra virgin oil or walnut oil

4 ounces farfalle pasta (whole wheat)

1 cup broccoli florets (small)

Method

Place water in large saucepan to boil.

Using a blender combine cayenne, pepper, salt, garlic and walnuts and then add lemon, parsley and broth until a creamy, smooth mixture is achieved.

Heat oil in medium size skillet over medium heat then put in chicken and stir until meat is cooked through.

Cook pasta in the boiling water and add bell pepper and broccoli and allow to cook while continuing to stir until the vegetables and pasta are tender then drain and return to pot. Add chicken and walnut sauce and toss.

Chopped Greek Salad with Chicken

This Greek inspired salad becomes a main course when chicken is added. Substitutions may be made with the vegetables so you can have cucumber or tomatoes or even bell peppers or broccoli.

Left over chicken may be used or some boneless chicken breasts can be poached or you can simply buy a roasted chicken. It can be served with hummus and pita bread.

Ingredients

2 tablespoons olive oil (extra-virgin)

⅓ cup red wine vinegar

1 teaspoon garlic powder

1 tablespoon fresh oregano or dill (chopped) or 1 teaspoon dried

¼ teaspoon salt

6 cups romaine lettuce (chopped)

¼ teaspoon pepper (freshly ground)

2 ½ cups cooked chicken (chopped)

2 chopped medium tomatoes

1 medium cucumber (chopped, seeded and peeled)

½ cup red onion (finely chopped)

½ cup feta cheese (crumbled)

½ cup ripe black olives (sliced)

Method

Whisk salt, pepper, garlic powder, vinegar, dill or oregano and oil in a bowl then add feta, olives, cucumber, onion, lettuce, cucumber, chicken and tomatoes. Toss until everything is well mixed. Serve.

Fish Couscous with Onion T'faya

This dish is served in Morocco for special occasions. This dish is known for its sweet, thick and heavily spiced sauce. This particular recipe is sweet and has a touch of sugar along with raisins which blends perfectly with the halibut.

Ingredients

4 tablespoons divided extra-virgin olive oil

½ cup raisins

2 tablespoons butter

2 teaspoons salt

8 threads saffron

1 teaspoon turmeric (ground)

1 teaspoon ginger (ground)

½ teaspoon nutmeg (ground)

½ teaspoon allspice (ground)

½ teaspoon pepper (freshly ground)

½ teaspoon cinnamon (ground)

1 tablespoon sugar

3 large thinly sliced onions

2 ½ pounds skinned Pacific halibut or other firm white fish (cut into pieces 2 inches wide)

2 ⅓ cups chicken broth, vegetable broth or fish broth

Freshly ground pepper (to taste)

½ cup slivered or sliced almonds

1 tablespoon canola oil

1 cup couscous (whole wheat)

Method

The raisins should be placed in a bowl and covered with warm water and allowed to soak for ten minutes.

Crush salt and saffron together to get a coarse powder then mix with pepper, cinnamon, nutmeg, turmeric, allspice and ginger in a bowl.

Heat two tablespoons of butter and olive oil in a heavy saucepan. Add the spices and stir until it starts foaming then add plumped raisins, sugar and onions. Keep stirring occasionally and cook until onions are slightly brown.

Add broth and place fish in onion mixture. Cook until fish is nice and flaky (*eight to ten minutes*). Takes off heat and season with some pepper then cover it and set it aside

In a small skillet heat some canola oil then add almonds and stir until they start to turn golden. When this is complete, place on paper towels to drain.

Bring the rest of the olive oil and broth to a boil in a saucepan the add couscous and stir. Cover, take it off the heat and let it stand for five minutes then fluff it using a fork.

When ready to serve make a mound of couscous on a shallow plate and top it with the fish and onion t'faya. Complete by sprinkling some almonds on top.

Apricot-Bulgur Pudding Cake with Custard Sauce

Just think of a rice pudding with bulgur. No matter what type of bulgur you choose to use when cooked it should look like cooked oatmeal.

Ingredients

⅓cup granulated sugar

½ cup dried apricots (chopped)

1 teaspoon orange zest (finely slivered)

1 cup water

1 cup freshly squeezed orange juice

½ cup bulgur

⅔ cup low-fat milk

2 large eggs (separated)

Custard Sauce

2 tablespoons brown sugar

½ cup toasted pistachios, (finely chopped & preferably salted)

Method

Using a saucepan combine water, orange juice, orange zest, sugar and apricots- bring to a boil then lower heat and cook while stirring until apricots are tender. Add bulgur and turn up heat allowing mix to come to a boil then reduce heat and simmer until bulgur is tender (*twenty minutes*).

Mixture should have consistency of cooked oatmeal. Then take off stove and allow to cool for ten minutes.

Place rack in center of oven and preheat to three hundred and fifty degrees Fahrenheit.

Whisk milk and egg yolks in bowl until well mixed then whisk in bulgur mixture slowly. Beat egg whites using mixer until peaks form and it is stiff. Add to bulgur mixture and fold in gently, using a metal spoon.

Place mixed batter in square eight inch baking dish. Add sugar to batter using a sieve to place evenly then place dish in roasting pan and put in oven. Hot water is to be placed in the roasting pan until water is half up the side of baking dish. Bake until cake is golden and puffed (half an hour to forty five minutes).

Remove dish from hot water and place on rack to cool to room temperature. Serve with custard sauce or cream and pistachios.

<u>Cherry Clafoutis</u>

Ingredients

1 pound pitted tart cherries, pitted

2 large eggs

⅓ cup plus ¼ cup sugar (divided)

2 tablespoons all-purpose flour

⅓ cup evaporated nonfat milk

1 ½ teaspoons vanilla extract

Confectioners' sugar (for dusting)

Method

Position rack in upper third of oven and preheat to three hundred and seventy five degrees. Coat nine inch shallow baking dish or glass quiche dish with cooking spray; mix one third cup sugar and cherries in dish then bake until cherries are juicy and tender (*twenty minutes*).

In the meantime whisk vanilla, flour and eggs with remaining sugar until you get a smooth mixture. Then whisk in evaporated milk.

Drain juice from cherries into a separate bowl. Spread cherries evenly in bowl then add egg mixture. Bake for twelve to fifteen

minutes until set. Use confectioners' sugar to dust and serve.
The cherry juice should be spooned over the top.

About The Author

Kara Milanova was hopping from diet to diet, trying to find the right one that would not only help her to lose weight but to live a healthier lifestyle as well. After a while she discovered the Mediterranean diet plan and soon realized that this was the way to go. She has even included a few of her favorite recipes as an added bonus.

Her main goal is to help those who are still on the fence about trying this diet to realize the benefits that they can accrue from changing their way of eating. She stresses that the Mediterranean diet is not really a diet but rather a lifestyle.

Kara knows that the main reason a lot of people find it extremely challenging to cut down on the consumption of animal products is because like her, they grew up eating these foods and are a little afraid of trying new ways especially with something as basic to their lives as food. She had emotional attachment to the foods she had grown up with and also many memories tied up with the food of childhood. Once Kara had decided to go for it she was encouraged to stay with the Mediterranean way of eating because she started to feel so much better in herself and had more energy. She is so happy about the change in her life that she wants to share it with everyone.